THE BLUE-GREEN SPEC

The healing powers of wild blue-green algae are truly broad-spectrum: among the conditions they have alleviated are dermatitis, obesity, heavy metal poisoning, depression, congestion, *Candida albicans* overgrowth, hypoglycemia and anemia. Dr. McKeith, who has improved her patients' health—and her own—with algae treatment, explains the makeup of this superfood and how to use it to optimize health.

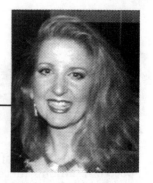

Gillian McKeith, Ph.D. is a practicing clinical nutritionist in the United Kingdom and Director of the McKeith Health Clinic of London. She conducts clinical research, publishes findings and treats illness through comprehensive nutritional biochemistry. Dr. McKeith incorporates orthomolecular nutrients, dietary counseling, allergy, toxic-metal and biochemical testing, and believes that most disease can be eradicated with the proper application of a natural and nutritional approach.

Dr. McKeith signed as the Healthy Living Expert for the BBC's "Good Morning Show" in Great Britain. She was the celebrity nutritionist for both the "Mike & Maty Show" on ABC and "The Joan Rivers Show." She also co-hosted the syndicated "Healthline Across America" radio program originating from Station WMCA in New York. Dr. McKeith authors regular editorial columns in national and international publications, and presents her "Ultimate Healthy Living" Workshops to audiences worldwide. She was educated at the University of Edinburgh, University of Pennsylvania, the London School of Acupuncture and the American Holistic College of Nutrition.

Miracle Superfood: Wild Blue-Green Algae

The nutrient powerhouse that stimulates the immune system, boosts brain power and guards against disease

Gillian McKeith, Ph.D.

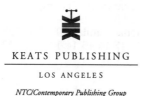

KEATS PUBLISHING

LOS ANGELES

NTC/Contemporary Publishing Group

Thank you

To my partner in life, dear Howard. Thank you from the heart of my soul for your encouragement, inspiration and special words. Your help has made it possible for me to share my algae story with others. It's a dream come true.

May you receive an abundance of Light. All my love, Gillian.

MIRACLE SUPERFOOD: WILD BLUE-GREEN ALGAE

Published by Keats
A division of NTC/Contemporary Publishing Group, Inc.
4255 West Touhy Avenue, Lincolnwood (Chicago), Illinois 60646-1975, U.S.A.
Copyright © 1999 by Gillian McKeith, Ph.D.
Printed and bound in the United States of America
International Standard Book Number: 0-87983-729-2
      04 RCP 18 17 16 15 14 13 12 11 10 9 8 7 6 5 4

Contents

ALGAE AND ME

As a clinical nutritionist, I have always prided myself on eating nutritious foods, exercising regularly and helping hundreds of my own clients to achieve optimum health. I had one secret blemish, however: small white specks appeared on my fingernails. Laboratory tests revealed my suspicions that I was deficient in the mineral zinc.

Zinc deficiency has been associated with infertility, hair-skin-nail problems, immune system dysfunction and various systemic disorders. Therefore, I attempted to supplement my intake of this vital mineral. Over the course of several years, I tried zinc capsules, tablets, lozenges and even zinc liquid. Nothing worked. My zinc deficiency persisted and my fingernails continued to be littered with the most awful white spots. It was obvious that my body was not absorbing the zinc supplements. Cognizant of the dangers of zinc deficiency (especially since I wanted to get pregnant), I kept my eyes open for other alternatives.

The revelation appeared at my doorstep several years ago; actually it occurred while I was cohosting a national health radio show in the U.S., "Healthline Across America." I was interviewing a guest who had survived an insidious strain of leukemia. After two relapses (a third relapse would be considered fatal) and chemotherapy radiation treatment, this patient had checked himself out of the hospital and turned his back on all of the conventional treatment that he claims were making him more ill. (Note: I would never condone a leukemic patient checking out of hospital.). Ten years later as a guest on my show, he was in the radio studio to tell us that he was now continually free of leukemia and feeling great. His horrifying disease had gone into remission. I asked him why he thought he was able to stave off a relapse for so long. He responded, "There's just one thing I'm doing differently." I countered, "What is that one thing?" He said, "I take something called blue-green algae from Klamath Lake every day, and I never miss taking it." At the time, I had never heard of this blue-green algae, but his words seemed to hit me like a ton of bricks.

I made it a point to find out all that I could about wild blue-green algae; it has now become my life-long obsession. I then began taking wild blue-green algae from Klamath Lake as part of my own nutritional regimen. Within 3 months, the white spots on my fingernails disappeared. I decided to take the blue-green algae all through my recent pregnancy as well. Every morning I made an algae drink which consisted of apple juice, aloe vera juice and water mixed with two teaspoons of the blue-green algae. Each time I drank this concoction, I felt as if my baby and womb were both expanding. The doctors were amazed when my petite frame produced a hefty eight-pound baby. I continued the wild blue-green algae drink after the birth. Many months later, I still continue to breast-feed; my gynecologist has said that I have the thickest creamiest mother's milk. I contribute much of my rapid recovery, my high energy level and my baby's wonderful development to this algae. I have since become one of the world's leading advocates of wild blue-green algae, specifically *Aphanizemenon flos-aqua* from Klamath Lake, Oregon.

WHAT ARE ALGAE?

A note on grammar. "Algae" is the plural of "alga," and is properly treated as a plural noun: "Algae are," etc. There are times, though, when this sounds awkward, and for my readers' and my own ease, I shall use the singular form when it is more comfortable: "Blue-Green algae is an excellent food." Now let us consider what algae are, or is.

Algae, also known as phytoplankton, are plant life without roots, leaves or flowers. It is estimated that there are more than 25,000 species of algae in existence. Most are mainly marine algae in the oceans; the rest are freshwater algae. Pond scums, water mosses, sea vegetables or seaweeds are all forms of algae. These algaes span an array of sizes from tiny picoplankton, which need to be magnified 1,000 times in order to be seen, to giant kelps in the oceans up to 50 meters in length. All algaes are composed of self-sufficient cells. For example, if you break off a piece, the broken piece and its host will still thrive. In addition, algaes can be separated by color. Algaes may be blue-green, green, red, brown, golden, purple. The deeper the color, the more intense is the spectrum of biochemical properties. The hot springs at Yellowstone National Park are called the "Paint Pots" because of the striking colors produced by the permanent residue of algae.

There are credible scientific and archaeological indications that during the first 30,000 years of the existence of our human race, algae were a significant source of food. The Aztec civilizations of ancient Mexico used and traded edible algae from their lakes. The algae were often mixed with maize (corn) to provide a nutritious meal. There is historical evidence to suggest that the ancient Incas of South America harvested and ate raw algae. And to this day the Kanembus tribe still eat algae from Lake Chad in Africa, just as their ancestors did; the algae are swept up with nets, sun-dried and shaped into small cakes, sold in the market at Chad's capital, N'Djamena and throughout the country. It is used for soups and sauces, like bouillon cubes. The algae-eating children of this tribe show no signs of malnutrition, unlike their non-algae eating neighbors, who suffer various degrees of malnutrition. Some scholars maintain that, in the Near East during biblical times, the food called manna was prepared with species of algae harvested from the Dead Sea. Moreover, red algae provided the name and color for the Red Sea.[1] For thousands of years, Chinese herbalists have been using algae to treat vitamin and mineral deficiencies. Algae are medically known in the Far East as an aid to digestion.

OXYGENATION

Algae have been around much longer than people, being in fact the initial form of life on Earth. Prior to the existence of algae, the Earth was a barren wasteland with only poisonous gases, devoid of oxygen. Algae assisted the process of making the environment habitable by animal life by using the power of the sun to split water molecules, combining the hydrogen part with carbon dioxide. This biochemical reaction allowed algae to create their own food from the surrounding gases and minerals. The oxygen half of the water molecule was freed into the atmosphere as a by-product, providing the basis for all human and animal life. To flourish, algae need only minerals, water and sunlight. Today, these remarkable forms of life are credited with up to 80 percent of nature's food supply and 90 percent of the Earth's oxygen production.[2] If there were no algae, life as we know it would cease to exist.

BLUE-GREEN ALGAE

Of all the many strains of different types of algae in existence, the blue-greens are the most distinct from other plants and algaes. There are anywhere form 500 to 1500 different species of these blue-green algaes.

Fossil records indicate that the blue-greens are the most primitive of all algaes, dating back over four billion years. These algaes have endured while thousands of other plant and animal species have become extinct.[3] The blue-greens are true survival pioneers, quickly changing and adapting to light conditions, temperatures and physical and chemical changes as the environment dictates.

They were probably the very first organisms to release elemental oxygen into the primitive and barren planetary atmosphere. In evolutionary terms, the blue-greens (scientifically known as Cyanobacteria) represent a link between bacteria and green plants.[4] This algae type, therefore, is both a plant and a healthy bacterium. Blue-green algae and bacteria have a similar composition. The genetic makeup, photosynthesis apparatus and the respiratory system are not separated by internal membranes. The "information" in the blue-green algae or bacteria, such as how to produce enzymes, how to digest antibiotics, how to repair cellular injury and how to quench free radicals is totally accessible. (Free radicals attack other molecules with which they come in contact.)

Blue-green algae and bacteria are sometimes referred to as prokaryotes (cells which lack membrane-bound nucleus). All other algaes and higher evolved plants are called eukaryotes. (The nucleus and pigments are confined within distinct membranes.) This is quite significant in terms of absorption, providing access to the goodness of the algae. Research scientist Daryl Kollman writes in his book *Hope Is a Molecule* about the ease of access to the nutrient profile: ". . . the essential bacteria in your intestinal tract [have] access to all the information contained in the blue-green algae." It is Kollman's opinion that "the biological information learned routinely by the blue-green algae" is information that the human race needs in order to survive. For instance, it might take us a million years to develop genetic information that would allow us to adapt to excess radiation; blue-green algae would adapt to it in a few months. When we eat the algae we then have access to that information and knowledge of adaptation to our surrounding environment, argues Kollman.

On a more metaphysical level, some algae enthusiasts believe that if you eat blue-green algae on a regular basis, you will connect with something essential and ancient. Richard France, a macrobiotic counselor, states, "It is not inconceivable that on subtle vibrational levels, unique genetic memories and messages of harmony and peace are stored in algae, which have grown undisturbed for aeons in a pristine environment. This information may be passed on to us at a cellular level, encouraging harmony among our own cellular family."

SHARED CHARACTERISTICS WITH PLANTS, ANIMALS, BACTERIA

Blue-green algae are quite distinct from other algaes in that they share characteristics with plants, animals and bacteria. Like plants, they have the ability to perform photosynthesis, but they do it far better than any other plant. They are the most chlorophyll-rich organisms on the planet.[5] Special phycolilin pigments initiate the conversion of light energy to chemical energy by certain wavelengths of visible light to which chlorophyll is not as sensitive. The energy is absorbed by the pohycolilins and passed onto the chlorophyll. Furthermore, blue-green algae are similar to animal cells in structure in that both have a soft, digestible cell wall composed of glycogen, which our bodies can use as a food. Many other plants have indigestible cellulose cell walls. Thus, because the algae's cell walls are soft and easy to digest, we can obtain more nutrients from its ingestion.

UNIQUENESS OF THE KLAMATH LAKE ALGAE STRAIN

Wild blue-green algae (*Aphanizemenon flos-aqua* or AFA) from Klamath Lake, Oregon is different and distinct from most algaes. It is a wild, uncultivated plant food. It is one of the few species of algae which grows wild in its own natural habitat, one of the world's most rich "nutrient traps." Unlike this indigenous and wild form of blue-green algae, some algaes are grown artificially in manmade farming ponds. The extraordinary and natural environment in which wild blue-green algae is grown is impossible to duplicate on these algae farms. Wild blue-green algae are completely free of artificial, synthetic influences. Because AFA is so purely and naturally grown in its own wild habitat, it has the most beneficial impact upon the human body. My basic argument is that wild AFA is superior: 1) in its rate of assimilability, digestibility and absorption, 2) as a food and energy source, 3) in nutrient density, and 4) as a preventative against disease.

Absorption

First, AFA algae have a soft cell glucose (glycoliprotein complex—protein bonded to carbohydrate) wall that is easily digested by the body; this allows rapid absorption and assimilation of vital nutrients. Other synthetically cultivated algaes and plants may have indigestible cellulose walls making absorption difficult or impossible. Wild blue-green algae is an anabolic substance. Translation: its organic compounds are more readily assimilated, absorbed, digested, metabolized and utilized by the human body.

Life Force Energy

Second, AFA algae require intense sunlight to grow. They favor the summer months in Oregon for their most prolific growth period. This may explain why they have such high levels of chlorophyll. Plant energy can be transferred from the chlorophyll directly to hemoglobin in the red blood cells of human blood plasma. The red blood cells and the plasma transfer the plant energy directly to the cells and to the bond structure, which then transmit it to the overall human body. AFA algae therefore have the ability to purify blood, quell inflammations and rejuvenate.

Fixing Nitrogen

Third, AFA is now known to fix nitrogen. This means that the algae breathe in nitrogen from the air to produce a rich source of proteins, nucleic acids, nitrogen compounds and other essential nutrients. These compounds enrich the soil and environment around them, as the nitrogen acts just like natural fertilizer. Unlike AFA, some algaes do not have the ability to metabolize nitrogen from the air and can only grow in soils where nitrogen compounds are already present or artificially added.

Nutrient Density

Fourth, AFA is a most nutrient-dense food with high concentrations of vitamins, minerals and other important natural substances. Over 95 percent of the nutrients can be used directly by the body in the same form. The vitamin B-complex profile of AFA is very high, especially vitamins B2, B6 and B12. For example, one gram of wild blue-green algae supplies more than the Recommended Daily Allowance (RDA) of vitamin B12. Vitamin B12 is essential for the production of red blood cells. It helps them to develop to a point where protein, folic acid, iron and vitamin C can mature properly and thus carry more oxygen to the cells. A deficiency of B12 may cause pernicious anemia. Restricted diets and poor absorption can cause a B12 deficiency. AFA has the highest active vegetable source of vitamin B12, in a form that is totally usable by the body. AFA algae have 65 times the B12 content of kelp, and almost 700 times more B12 than alfalfa. The B vitamins within AFA algae are of such high quality that they can boost the body's energy level, endurance and stamina. B vitamins convert carbohydrates into glucose, which the body can then utilize to produce energy. The ability of blue-green algae to efficiently transfer glucose into energy (via the B vitamins) may represent its most important health contribution.

In addition, the algae strain AFA has a broader spectrum of minerals than any other green algae. To date, over 40 macro- and microminerals have been identified in the wild blue-green algae.[6] These minerals are bound into a colloidal matrix, which means they are enzyme-bound. Such configurations cannot be synthesized. Choline, an ingredient important to the brain's phospholipids, is absent in many blue-greens but is present in AFA algae. AFA is an elixir for the brain unlike any other algae and has a beneficial impact upon brain synchronization: it specifically enhances the hypothalamus, the pineal and pituitary glands. In my own clinical research, I have found patients reporting improved mental clarity, enhanced memory and a sharper sense of focus after ingesting AFA algae for several months. It ought to be noted that AFA has a slightly bitter taste. According to traditional Chinese medicine, bitter flavors influence the heart-mind system, actually helping the mind to focus better. Victor Kubinskas in his book *Survival into the 21st Century* described it as a "mental buzz and blissed out feeling." You can't achieve this type of mind enhancement with any other algae.

AFA has a much higher concentration of vitamin C than any other algae. This is important because iron needs the synergistic effect of vitamin C to be properly assimilated in our bodies. The iron content of wild blue-green algae is equally impressive; its ability to build the quality of the blood is thus superior. Of its dry weight, more than two-thirds of AFA is assimilable protein, more than any other algae. AFA wild blue-green algae gets its protein content from atmospheric nitrogen. AFA may even have "special vibrational fields." Dr. Gabriel Cousins describes it as "subtle, organized energy fields." These vibrational energy fields are the life forces of the algae, which he believes has the ability to regenerate mind, body and immune forces.[7] Therefore, more so than any other algae, this wild blue-green strain is a perfect food and perfect food supplement in preventing and treating nutritional deficiencies, imbalances or disorders.

Please note that when I refer to "wild blue-green algae," I mean specifically the Aphanizemenon flos-aqua (AFA) strain. I use the terms interchangeably, the only difference being that one is the biochemical name and the other the common name.

THE ALGAE OF KLAMATH LAKE

Klamath Lake is one of the world's richest sources of the AFA strain of wild blue-green algae, the strain scientifically referred to as Aphanizemenon flos aqua (AFA). This lake is nestled 3000 feet up in the almost inaccessible Cascade Mountains of Oregon, boasting one of the most abundant supplies of minerals and trace elements. This mineral treasury is the result of massive volcanic eruptions that occurred several thousand years ago, blanketing the area with millions of tons of mineral-rich volcanic ash. Fifty thousand tons of this ash flow every day into the 140-square mile lake from the 4000-square mile volcanic basin through a network of 17 rivers, streams and falls. This spectacular lake in its unique position of isolation has become a natural power-packed nutrient-trap impossible for man to duplicate. The blue-green algae from Klamath Lake grows wild; it is free of adverse bacteria, heavy metals, pesticides, herbicides, insecticides and fungicides.[8]

TOXICITY

Algae researcher Dr. William Barry has personally examined many blooms of the AFA strain from Klamath Lake (and other lakes too) and has never found any toxicity.[9] A research report produced by Rapala in *The Journal of Applied Phycology* (1993) confirmed Barry's conclusion; this report emphatically states that the AFA algae strain is not capable of producing toxins. As further testament to its safety, it should be noted that hundreds of thousands of people worldwide have consumed the AFA strain algae with no trace of toxicity.[10] The only time that AFA should be used cautiously is when you are extremely weak, thin, very dry with a *cold* constitution or are already pregnant.

There are two strains of blue-green algae which have produced toxins at various times: one is called *Anaboena-flos aquae*, the other *Microcystic aeroginosa*. Neither strain is produced commercially and so human consumption would be virtually impossible. The focus of this book is on the nontoxic and safe AFA wild blue-green strain, rather than any potentially toxic forms.

NUTRITIONAL CONTENT

AFA wild blue-green algae is the most nutrient-dense and perfectly balanced whole food in the world. With a dynamic nutritional profile, it is the richest source of almost every nutrient in its purest form. Because it is recognized by the body as a food, it is immediately available with a greater than 90 percent assimilation rate. This means that the body is capable of utilizing virtually all of the algae's nutrients. When taking a conventional multiple vitamin with minerals, the body may only absorb a small fraction of the actual nutrient dosages. In my own clinical practice, I tell my patients that what you eat is important; but what you absorb and assimilate may even be more important.

AFA blue-green algae has an extraordinarily high content of vitamins, minerals, amino acids (complete protein) and live enzymes: including a complete amino acid profile with 62 percent protein content, high in beta-carotene, antioxidants and the highest known natural dietary source of vitamin B12 and chlorophyll.

The nutritional composition of the foods we eat is vital, as it determines just how much energy our bodies need to break down and process those foods. The more processed the food, the harder our bodies have to work. The more cooked-out foods we eat, the more strain we place on our enzyme quotient. Enzymes are protein molecules which digest our food and make it small enough to pass through the minute pores of the intestines into the blood. Modern diets are so devoid of key nutrients and enzymes to help break foods down and absorb their goodness that we tire our bodies from simple food abuse. This is why you may feel tired after meals, or bloated and low in energy.

Extra energy is needed to break down and absorb foods that are "empty" or nutrient deficient. Further energy is required to break down and eliminate pesticides and other toxins from our food and environment, and to curb the disruptive effects of high levels of mental stress. The end result is low energy and poor elimination of toxins and waste products. Our bodies then store these nasty residues in our fat cells, in the bloodstream and in the key organs. We poison ourselves and rob our bodies of strength. Depletion of energy reserves is thought to contribute to the fall in immunity and the rise in degenerative diseases that we are now witnessing.

MINERALS

One of the greatest contributions of blue-green AFA algae is its full spectrum of minerals. Minerals are the framework for our bodies, critical to our overall mental and physical well-being. Bones, teeth, muscle, blood, nerve cells, tissues and internal fluids all contain varying quantities of minerals. They help to build the skeletal structure, regulate the heart, balance internal pressure of body fluids, nerve response and oxygen transport from the lungs to the tissues. Minerals act as catalysts for many biological reactions within the body, including muscle response, digestion, metabolism of nutrients in foods, and transmission of messages through the nervous system. Minerals help to maintain the body's delicate water balance, allowing the mental and physical processes to function properly. They keep blood and tissue fluids from becoming too acid or too alkaline, thus balancing the body's pH. Minerals permit other nutrients to pass into the bloodstream. Minerals also help draw chemical substances in and out of the cells and aid in the creation of antibodies. The problem with minerals, however, is that they can only be supplied to the human body through diet.[11] Thus, if your diet is poor, your mineral profile will be poor, too. Not only are we often robbed of minerals by our inadequate diets, but most soils in which our produce grows are severely mineral deficient. Remember, your body cannot make minerals: if they are not in the soil, they are not in the produce, and are certainly not in you.

A U.S. government paper illustrated this problem forcefully when leading authorities from Johns Hopkins University, Yale, Columbia University and the U.S. Department of Agriculture reported that "Ninety-nine percent of the American people are deficient in food complexed minerals. A marked deficiency in any one of the more important minerals actually results in

Table 1. Mineral Content of AFA Algae

1 gram of AFA algae provides the following minerals:

Boron	14.0 mcg	Molybdenum	3.30 mcg
Calcium	12.70 mg	Nickel	5.3 mcg
Chloride	0.47 mg	Phosphorus	5.20 mg
Chromium	0.53 mcg	Potassium	12.00 mcg
Cobalt	2.00 mcg	Selenium	0.67 mcg
Copper	4.30 mcg	Silicon	186.70 mcg
Fluoride	38.00 mcg	Sodium	2.70 mg
Germanium	0.27 mcg	Tin	0.47 mcg
Iodine	0.53 mcg	Titanium	23.3 mcg
Iron	0.37 mg	Vanadium	2.70 mcg
Magnesium	2.20 mg	Zinc	18.70 mcg
Manganese	32.0 mcg		

Figures listed are average figures only. Precise nutritional amounts may vary depending on the algae batch.

disease. Any upset of the balance, any considerable lack of one or another element, however microscopic the body requirement may be, can cause us to sicken, suffer and shorten our lives."[12] And that statement was issued in the 1930s! The matter has worsened since then. Therefore, I propose that AFA blue-green algae can potentially prevent, correct, alleviate and treat these mineral imbalances and deficiencies.

Trace minerals or microminerals are needed in minute quantities by the body. No one mineral can function without affecting the others. Each mineral needs other minerals for proper utilization. For example, calcium requires magnesium for its absorption and assimilation. Moreover, a deficiency of even just one mineral can cause severe imbalances of vitamins as well.

In my own practice, blood tests have revealed that 98 percent of the people who first come to see me are deficient in one or more macro- or micromineral. More troubling, the pregnant women who have come to my office were all deficient in certain minerals on their first visit. I correct these mineral deficiencies with algae, and other components if necessary. Getting enough minerals in the right balance is critical if you are to feel well; wild blue-green algae seems to provide a framework for a perfect mineral balance.

Wild blue-green algae contains all the essential trace minerals: boron, calcium, chromium, cobalt, copper, iron, magnesium, manganese, phosphorus, potassium, sodium, zinc and vanadium. Since the algae is in such a natural state, it is conceivable that it may even contain other minerals not yet discovered or identified. But the most significant story here is that these minerals are in perfect balance for maximum benefits and positive impact upon human biochemistry.

In my practice, the most common mineral deficiency I have discovered is magnesium. Magnesium is an essential part of many digestive systems and metabolic processes. According to studies, 80 to 90 percent of the US population may be deficient in the mineral magnesium.[13] Dr. Mildred Seelig, one of the country's leading authorities on magnesium (along with Dr. William Rea) suggests also that approximately 90 percent of the population is magnesium deficient.[14] I have been able to correct magnesium deficiencies using AFA wild blue-green algae.

As I mentioned at the outset, I suffered for years with a zinc deficiency, even though I was ingesting zinc supplements. Zinc is an essential trace mineral required by the body in larger amounts than any other trace mineral except iron. It is an essential cofactor needed by more than 100 enzymes in the eyes, liver, kidneys, muscles, skin, bones, testes and other organs.[15] To maintain plasma zinc concentrations, frequent intakes of dietary zinc are necessary.[16] Zinc is critical in maintaining many healthy bodily organs and functions. The blue-green AFA algae finally corrected my zinc deficiency only because the mineral composition of the algae was perfectly balanced and bioavailable, thus allowing my body efficient absorption and assimilation of this key mineral.

According to Dr. Maurice Schiff, a Professor of Medicine at the University of California at San Diego, the extraordinary mineral profile of the algae will combine and arrange its mineral matrix as if it were identical to the building blocks of our own flesh. "Because everything is in its proper proportion, it is readily absorbed by the body,"[17] he concludes. It is worth noting that wild blue-green algae has one of the highest sources of cobalt, the essential mineral part of vitamin B12 and one of the highest natural concentrations of iron known. The AFA thus builds up the quality of our blood and assists in resistance to infection and diseases.

VITAMINS

Wild blue-green algae contains the most perfect balance of vitamins of all algaes. Vitamins are essential to life. They aid in digestion, elimination and resistance to disease. Depletions or deficiencies can lead to various nutritional disorders, depending on which vitamins may be lacking in the diet. With a few exceptions, most vitamins cannot be manufactured by the body. They must be supplied by the diet or by supplement pills. The vitamin composition of blue-green algae is far superior to any multivitamin supplement pills. In a recent study at Yale New Haven Hospital 257 brands of multivitamin supplement pills were evaluated. The study concluded that 80 percent of the vitamin pills were inadequate, incomplete or imbalanced.[18] With wild-blue green algae, the composition and balance of vitamins is in perfect harmony with human biochemistry for maximum utilization.

Table 2. Key Vitamins in AFA Algae

B1	(thiamine)	choline
B2	(riboflavin)	pantothenic acid (B5)
B6	(pyridoxine)	biotin
B3	(niacin)	folic acid
B12		E
C	(ascorbic acid)	

PROTEINS/AMINO ACIDS

Wild blue-green AFA algae is an exceptionally high source of protein (60 percent), nearly identical to the human body's protein composition. The quality of the protein in AFA algae is superior to that of most other plant or animal protein sources, being derived from all eight essential amino acids. It is important for general good health of the skin, hair, nails, brain, ligaments, bones, teeth, hormones, sex glands and enzymes that we eat foods with all eight essential amino acids. If even one amino acid is missing, then the body cannot make protein. Because plant proteins tend to lack certain amino acids, some vegetarians may suffer from a deficiency of basic protein. On the other hand, meats (including fish, chicken, beef, turkey) usually contain all eight essential amino acids to form complete protein. But studies clearly indicate that animal protein raises cholesterol, increases the risk of heart disease and forms excess mucus. In addition, animal protein is rather difficult to digest. If protein digestion is incomplete, then bacteria can form toxic compounds. AFA algae protein is of a type called glycoprotein, whereas meat and regular vegetable protein is of a type called lipoprotein. The body must convert lipoproteins into glycoproteins in order to utilize it. Since algae is already in the form of glycoprotein, the body need not make any biochemical conversion. Thus, eating the blue-green algae protein is more biochemically efficient and preserves metabolic energy. The protein in AFA algae is 85 percent assimilable, compared to beef with just a 20 percent assimilable rate.[19] Improper or incomplete protein digestion may not only produce toxins, but may very well render the protein worthless.

Finally, AFA protein assists in nourishing the brain and nervous system because of algae's rich source of amino acid peptides. These peptides are precursor for neurotransmitters which carry messages from the brain to ordinary muscles, and from the organs back to the brain. Although the brain comprises just two percent of total body weight, it actually uses 20 percent of the body's energy resources. Thus, the brain needs to be fed and satisfied virtually every minute of the day. The nervous system and brain interface with each other continually as messages are sent back and forth incessantly. Therefore, if there is the slightest break in this amino acid-peptide link, you may experience memory loss, mental fatigue or nervous disorders.

ENZYMES

There are thousands of live active enzymes in AFA algae. Enzymes are critical for life; they are the body's labor force. Enzymes metabolize, digest and assimilate all substances entering the body. For example, live enzymes digest food, destroy toxins, even break down fats and cellulose and metabolize starch and proteins. Furthermore, enzymes are involved in moving muscles, nourishing nerves, stimulating brain function, breathing, accompanying male sperm and female eggs, fighting off illness, infection and disease and more. A shortage of live active enzymes could wreak havoc in your body.

Unfortunately, most people do not have sufficient enzyme activity. Although the pancreas manufactures a certain limited number of enzymes for digestion, there is still a need to sup-

Table 3. Amino Acid Content of AFA Algae

Essential	Semiessential	Nonessential
Isolelucine	Arginine	Alanine
Leucine	Histidine	Aspartic Acid
Lysine		Cystine
Methionine		Glutamic Acid
Tryptophan		Proline
Threonine		Serine
Phenylalanine		Tyrosine
Valine		

plement the body with additional enzymes.[20] Supplementary enzymes are generally acquired through the foods that we eat; raw fruits and vegetables are packed with live active enzymes. However, these supplementary enzymes are easily destroyed when we cook, broil, boil, bake, fry, sauté, poach or even freeze our foods. The enzymes within the body are further destroyed by stress, fatigue, chemical pollutants, even pregnancy and possibly an extraordinarily strenuous exercise regime. Thus, the thousands of live active enzymes within wild blue-green AFA algae can contribute to a substantially healthier life.

PIGMENTS

Wild blue-green algae is rich in all kinds of botanical pigments. A pigment is a molecule capable of absorbing wavelengths of light, and then reflecting it as a recognizable color.

Chlorophyll

A prominent pigment is chlorophyll, the green substance of plants. Wild blue-green algae is a higher source of cholorophyll than any other plant or algae. Chlorophyll is the lifeblood of AFA algae. It is similar in molecular structure to heme, the oxygen carrying red pigment of human blood. However, chlorophyll contains magnesium at its cell center, whereas blood contains iron. Chlorophyll within the algae is a powerful oxygenator for human beings. And without sufficient oxygen, we can develop symptoms of low energy, sluggish digestion and low metabolism. Dr. Otto Warburg, the 1931 Nobel Prize winner for physiology and medicine, concluded that oxygen deprivation was a major cause of cancer.[21]

In the early 20th century, chlorophyll was regarded as a crucial weapon against various common health complaints. Many physicians used it in the treatment of pain relief, skin disorders, ulcers and even as a breath freshener. However, after World War II, chlorophyll was replaced by chemical antiseptics. Today there is a renewed interest in chlorophyll.

This renewed interest is certainly justified. Chlorophyll's health benefits are indeed numerous: helping the body to obtain more oxygen, aiding digestion, acting as an anti-inflammatory, healing gum disease, preventing infection, minimizing the effects of pollution and accelerating wound healing. Chlorophyll can be ingested to combat bad breath and body odor, acting like an internal deodorant for your inner organs. According to biochemist Lita Lee, Ph.D., "Chlorophyll appears to stimulate the regeneration of damaged liver cells, and increases circulation to all organs by dilating blood vessels. In the heart, chlorophyll aids in the transmission of nerve impulses that control contraction. The heart rate is slowed, yet each contraction is increased in power, improving the efficiency of cardiac power." [22]

AFA's chlorophyll also helps to balance alkalinity, thereby reducing acidity in the body. Stress, excess protein and fat in a diet can make your body acidic. When your system becomes even slightly acidic, free radical formation and oxidative damage increase, thus raising the risk of disease. According to Dr. Julian Whitaker, "A more serious consequence of acidity is that it causes calcium to be mobilized out of your bones to buffer the acid and make you more alkaline. The slightly acidic condition brought on by eating too much protein is a primary reason we have such widespread osteoporosis. The calcium that is mobilized from the bone to buffer or neutralize this excessive acidity is lost in the urine." Dr. Whitaker believes that eating blue-green algae, with its high chlorophyll content, is a natural and effective way to correct this excess acidity.[23]

Phycocyanins
Wild blue-green algae contains a host of other pigments, including phycocyanins. Phycocyanin is the pigment which gives wild blue-green algae its blue hue; it is a protein which has been shown to inhibit the formation of cancer colonies.[24] These various pigments operate in the body with the human pigment bilirubin to keep the liver functioning at optimum capacity, and aid in the digestion of amino acids. Phycocyanin helps draw together amino acids for neurotransmitter formation, which may increase mental capacity. These special pigments contribute to the proper functioning of other metabolic processes as well.

RNA/DNA

Wild blue-green algae contains approximately 4 percent RNA/DNA. The RNA/DNA (nucleic acids) is needed by the body to make new cells, repair damaged cells and for growth of body tissue. As we get older, the levels of RNA/DNA decrease. If you do not have enough RNA/DNA, you may suffer the consequences of a weak immune system and ultimately age prematurely. Inferior eating habits, pollution and stress can deplete your RNA/DNA quotient. Keeping RNA/DNA levels at a consistent level is therefore important if you want to retard cell destruction, enhance immunity and regenerate your body. Eating wild blue-green algae will supply more of this RNA/DNA to your body.

LIPIDS

Lipids, sometimes interchangeably called essential fatty acids (what I call the healthy fats), are highly represented in wild blue-green algae. These lipids are critical for life itself and provide the most concentrated source of energy for the body. Fatty acids function as carriers for vitamins A, E and K, and are important for the conversion of plant beta-carotene into vitamin A. These lipids nourish the nerves and blood vessels, and lubricate skin and tissues. Thus, lipids within AFA can prevent the skin and other bodily tissues from becoming dry and scaly.[24] The omega-3 and omega-6 essential fatty acids (EPA and gamma-linolenic acid) are known to help prevent heart disease, reduce serum cholesterol and raise HDL (good) cholesterol.

BETA-CAROTENE

Wild blue-green algae is one of the highest known natural sources of beta-carotene; its rich levels of chlorophyll contribute to the outstanding beta-carotene content. Within the wild blue-green algae, the chlorophyll and beta-carotene work together. The chlorophyll activates enzymes which produce vitamins E and K. These vitamins help to convert the carotene into vitamin A. An advantage of using the beta-carotene from algae as a source of vitamin A is its nontoxic property. When green food containing beta-carotene is ingested, it is converted into vitamin A in the liver as the body needs it, whereas vitamin A from animal products is potentially toxic in very large doses. Wild blue-green algae, due to its high chlorophyll content, will convert more than twice as much carotene into vitamin A as would other foods.[25] You can obtain relatively high amounts of immune-boosting beta-carotene when ingesting relatively small amounts of algae.

Wild blue-green algae's beta-carotene is a powerful antioxidant and anti-infective protector against skin disorders, night blindness, environmental pollutants, allergies, ageing and immune system dysfunction. Twenty-five years of worldwide research confirm that people who ingest foods high in beta-carotene have a lower incidence of lung, stomach, colon, bladder, uterus, ovary and skin cancers.[26]

AFA is one of the few foods containing both forms of beta-carotene, the cis form and the trans form. (Synthetic beta-carotene found in supplements and root vegetables is of the trans form, fruits and vegetables consist of the cis form.) When both forms are eaten together, the absorption rate of the beta-carotene can be over 10 times that of just the trans form by itself. [27]

COMPLEX CARBOHYDRATES

The complex carbohydrates found in wild blue-green algae are readily usable by our bodies. The algae's carbohydrate content is immediately available for conversion to energy. Carbohydrates are the main source of energy for all bodily functions.

NUTRITIONAL BENEFITS

Almost 98 percent of the patients I see in my clinical practice are deficient in one or more minerals or vitamins. Yet our health is dependent on complete availability and absorption of nutrients in a form that our bodies can utilize. Even a deficiency in just one nutrient can cause a chain reaction, triggering deficiencies in many other nutrients. There are many biochemical and nutritional reasons for poor nutrient absorption which may include (1) a sluggish body, (2) excess of unhealthy mucus along the walls of the small intestines, (3) nutrient-deficient foods, (4) malfunctioning digestive system.

It is possible that a person may consistently take vitamin or mineral supplement pills, with little or no recognized benefit if the body's biochemical absorption system fails to function properly. Unlike supplement pills and unlike most other foods, the AFA algae has a greater than 90 percent assimilation rate. This means that the algae, recognized by the body as a food, absorbs with unsurpassed efficiency and rapidity when compared to most other natural or perhaps unnatural substances. Thus, even if a person's internal absorption system is malfunctioning, the algae is so biologically assimilable that tangible benefits can still be obtained nonetheless. For these reasons, the wild blue-green algae could play a major role in wiping out malnutrition. For example, an acclaimed study on severely malnourished children, under the auspices of the Central American University (1994), found that 79 percent of these subjects no longer exhibited nutritional symptoms of malnutrition after just six months on the algae.[28] In addition, NASA has been studying the algae as a possible food source for space missions.[29] It is understandable that this algae delivers such a broad spectrum of nutritional benefits ranging from weight loss to memory booster to immune system enhancer and much more; it's all in the rate of assimilation and absorption. Finally, it's interesting to note that the Russians have used algae to treat patients exposed to radiation in the Chernobyl nuclear disaster.[30]

Following are summaries of this algae's potential nutritional benefits, based on my own clinical research and clinical case studies and other research reports as well.

MALABSORPTION

It has often been said that you are what you eat. You are not. In reality, you are really what you digest and absorb. You can eat what you might think are nutritious, high-quality foods, and ingest the best nutritional supplement pills, but if you do not digest and absorb what you consume, you will not enjoy the benefits of optimal health. Incomplete or faulty digestive processes may lead to a wide variety of chronic disorders. It has been suggested that 80 percent of diseases might be caused by improperly digested foods and their toxic by-products being absorbed into the body. Signs of poor nutrient absorption can include bloating, flatulence, indigestion, hair loss, diarrhea, constipation, muscle fatigue, allergies and even mood swings.

In my own clinical research, I have found that AFA wild blue-green algae helps to correct malabsorption and ultimately malnutrition. For example, tests at my clinic, the McKeith Health Clinic of London, have revealed extensive deficiencies in many individuals of every important mineral. Yet minerals need to be present for the body to function at optimum capacity. After prescribed regimens of AFA algae, most if not all minerals are significantly elevated, usually to normal range. I have been unable to achieve such results using isolated mineral supplement pills. In other cases where patients may suffer from excesses of certain minerals, the algae has often corrected these imbalances too. It seems that AFA algae has the ability to achieve balance for the body's biochemistry.

Clinical Case Study: Mrs. Simmons, Patient, 62
Mrs. Simmons complained of low energy, splitting nails, indigestion and hair loss. She worried about osteoporosis. She could not exercise because she simply had "no energy."

Various tests at our clinic revealed the following about Mrs. Simmons:

First Visit		After 4 months		After 8 months	
Lead	High	Lead	Lower still not normal	Lead	Normal
Calcium	Low	Calcium	Low, but improved	Calcium	Normal
Magnesium	Low	Magnesium	Low, but improved	Magnesium	Normal
Chromium	Low	Chromium	Normal	Chromium	Normal
Zinc	Low	Zinc	Normal	Zinc	Normal
Selenium	Low	Selenium	Normal	Selenium	Normal
Iron	Low	Iron	Normal	Iron	Normal
Vanadium	Low	Vanadium	Normal	Vanadium	Normal

The algae program started out at 1 gram daily, building up to 10 grams, then reducing to 2 grams. Mrs. Simmons maintains her mineral levels using liquid algae of 4 drops daily. The first change she noticed was increased energy levels. She says she "never knew what energy was until using blue-green algae." Cerebral stimulus is also noticeable. Mrs. Simmons says she "thinks more clearly and remembers detail better."

Comment: Initially, Mrs. Simmons showed low levels of calcium, the most needed mineral in our bodies. Calcium is required for various body processes such as nerve and muscle actions, metabolism of Vitamin D, and for the health of bones and teeth. It is extremely difficult to absorb calcium, however, as most people can often only assimilate no more than 20 percent-30 percent of ordinary calcium supplements. But the calcium contained in wild blue-green algae is fully absorbable and assimilable.[31]

Clinical Case Study: Dorothy, Patient, 35
Since age 17, after a bout of glandular fever, Dorothy had continual fingernail problems: the nails have been brittle, covered in white spots and chip easily. This condition is known as leukonykia, and is often linked with a zinc deficiency and malabsorption. At 35 years of age, Dorothy arrived at my clinic complaining that the nail problem had accelerated and was now accompanied by excessive hair loss.

Blood tests and hair mineral analysis revealed low levels of B12, folate, and zinc. Over the years Dorothy had tried all types of nutrients including multimineral complexes, the B vitamins and four different types of zinc (liquid, capsule, tablet and lozenge). Dorothy was amazed to find out through my blood tests and hair analysis that she was still zinc deficient after all these years of supplementation. She simply was not absorbing zinc and other nutrients and minerals. Zinc absorption may vary from about 20–40 percent of ingested zinc.

Dorothy's Algae Program

Weeks 1 & 2: ½ teaspoon daily (½ gram)
Weeks 3 & 4: 1 teaspoon daily (1 gram)
Weeks 5–8: 2 teaspoons daily (2 grams)
Weeks 8–12: 2 heaping teaspoons daily (4 grams)
Weeks 13–16: 2 heaping teaspoons twice daily (8 grams)
Weeks 17–21: decreased dosage to 2 teaspoons daily (2 grams)
Patient is now on a maintenance of 1 teaspoon per day (1 gram).

After six weeks on my program of algae, Dorothy's white spots on the fingernails had started to diminish. After 16 weeks, the white spots had disappeared completely; the hair was no longer falling out. The patient also claims to have more energy and recently became pregnant after 4 years of failed attempts.

Comment: Although Dorothy was ingesting different forms of zinc for years, she was obviously not absorbing this important mineral. Deficiency of zinc is associated with the maintenance of body tissues, sexual function, reproductive system, immunity and detoxification. Research now shows that zinc is probably involved in more body functions than any other mineral. Although the dosages of the various nutrients in the algae are relatively low, the absorption rate and the body's ability to metabolize it are outstanding.

BURPS, GAS, BLOATING

Burps, gas, wind, flatulence, nausea, feeling of heaviness, diarrhea, watery stools, constipation, irritable bowel and indigestion are all signs of what I call the "body plumbing backing up." AFA wild blue-green algae can be a big help in correcting these types of problems.

Clinical Case Study: Mr. Richards, Patient, 46
Six months ago, Mr. Richards came to the McKeith Health Clinic. Patient complained of constant bloating, gas and wind. These symptoms were often accompanied by nausea, diarrhea and indigestion. Mr. Richards had some excess flab, felt tired and lacked motivation. He had grown up on a meat-and-potatoes diet with lots of dairy products and refined, processed foods.

I immediately started him on wild blue-green algae, a teaspoon before each meal. He desperately needed more digestive enzymes, of which there are hundreds in wild blue-green algae. Stool tests showed that he was suffering from pancreatic insufficiency and an imbalance of healthy flora. This means that the pancreas, the organ which makes enzymes to digest food, is exhausted. Thus, enzymes are not produced in sufficient quantities, and fail to reach the stomach and intestines where digestion should take place. End result: nutrients are not absorbed.

In addition, Mr. Richards ate mainly cooked foods. Cooking food destroys all the digestive enzymes. I selected the blue-green algae because of its bitter action. It is this action that can improve digestion substantially, since the bitterness stimulates your taste buds, activates the membranes of the gastrointestinal tract and encourages the nerves of your body to produce more secretions to aid digestion; nutrients from the foods you eat can therefore be absorbed better. Wild blue-green algae provided Mr. Richards with more than adequate levels of active enzymes, B6, zinc and other essential B vitamins which also help to stimulate production of these important food-digesting enzymes. Mr. Richards followed my recommendation of combining his foods correctly to maximize digestion (i.e., fruit alone, separate starches and proteins). After 6 months, Mr. Richards is bloat and gas free. Follow-up stool tests reveal healthy intestinal flora and normal pancreas activity. A side effect of all his efforts . . . he lost just about 30 pounds in weight.

MEMORY BOOSTER

Wild blue-green algae has benefited many patients complaining of poor memory or lack of concentration. This is most likely due to the high usable protein content and large number of neuropeptides (brain transmitters) which cross the blood-brain barrier. The intense supply of nutrients present in the algae may nourish weakened nerves, and thus improve brain function and memory. The Central American University Report (1994) on malnourished grammar school children stated that academic results and exam scores improved dramatically after trials of wild blue-green algae.[28]

In *The Journal of Orthomolecular Medicine* (1985), Dr. Gabriel Cousins reported positive effects of wild blue-green algae on brain function in both of two closely-followed patients. Each patient had been diagnosed with Alzheimer's, a degenerative disease of the brain. Dr. Cousins says that he "personally witnessed brain function enhancing qualities" in both individuals. One 66-year-old woman, with a seven-year history of the disease, showed a partial reversal of her symptoms after six months on wild blue-green algae. She could communicate better, watch television, understand what was happening and even dress herself. Her spirit, humor and sense of awareness improved dramatically. There was no change in long-term memory, but short-term memory had significantly increased. The second patient, a 64-year-old lawyer, suffering for three years with Alzheimer's, was "rapidly going downhill," reports Cousins, until the senile degeneration was arrested using wild blue-green algae. Dr. Cousins suggests that it "may be possible to temporarily halt the progression of Alzheimer's disease, to partially reverse it or even help to prevent it." It would, however, take a comprehensive study to make possible any definitive statements about the effects of wild blue-green algae on Alzheimer's disease.

Dr. Cousins further points out in his book *Spiritual Nutrition and the Rainbow Diet* that "Aphanizemenon flos-aqua algae seems to activate mind-brain function in about 70–80 percent of those who use it." In my own clinical practice, nearly every patient who is using the wild blue-green algae reports to me that they can perform more mental work for longer periods, and that memory ultimately improves. Medical researcher Tom Warren, in his book *Beating Alzheimer's*, writes that wild blue-green algae is an integral part of his nutrient program. Warren argues that Alzheimer's patients do not have enough protein in their brains. The protein in wild blue-green algae is of a high quality and fully assimilable. AFA algae also contains choline, the "brain enhancing" B vitamin. According to Sherry Rogers, M.D., manganese deficiency is one of the potential causes of presenile brain degradation; wild blue-green algae can correct and prevent a manganese deficiency. Finally, the internationally renowned orthomolecular researcher Abram Hoffer has emphatically stated that most cases of true senility are the result of prolonged and subtle nutritional deficiencies.

Clinical Case Study: Mary, Patient, 16

You don't need to be suffering from Alzheimer's disease to be in need of a memory booster. When Mary came to the McKeith Health Clinic, she was suffering from short-term memory difficulties, confusion and concentration problems. Mary was studying for university entrance exams. Mock exams showed her grades were lower than they used to be; average, but not good enough for the university. Mary's teachers all knew that she was not performing to her true aptitude levels. Patient told me she simply had no mental energy for study. Other symptoms included headaches, skin problems, frequent infections, a general feeling of being unwell, and stress. Normally a high achiever, Mary was burning the candles at both ends with extracurricular school activities. Performance declined in those activities as well.

Blood analysis indicated low calcium, magnesium, zinc and vanadium. Amino acid profile revealed several key amino acids to be borderline low. Urine tests indicated low-grade viral infection and acid-alkaline imbalance. I started Mary on a wild blue-green algae program of tablets. She started out slowly on only 1 gram tablet daily. I did not want to overwhelm her as she had never taken a nutrient supplement in her life. I slowly built the tablet dosage up to 4 a day over a 4-week period. Over the next 2 months, this was doubled to 4 tablets twice daily. She implemented some of my dietary recommendations, along with additional digestive enzyme support.

Mary just took her final exams. She told me that her grades have "gone up dramatically." She has "clarity of mind." The "bowels are moving regularly and [her] headaches have gone away." Mary says her skin is smoother. A final bonus: Mary told me that her menstrual periods used to be painful and heavy since the age of 13; her periods are now lighter and pain-free.

Comment: Painful menstruation can often be linked to low calcium, magnesium and essential fatty acids. Excessive menstrual bleeding is often caused by a stagnant liver. These imbalances can often be corrected using wild blue-green algae along with other nutritional support. The brain enhancement was most likely the end result of the high number of neuropeptides in the algae. Wild blue-green algae is a neurostimulant, and is therefore, able to abundantly feed the pathways to the brain cells.

IMPROVE IMMUNE SYSTEM

Too many people today suffer the consequences of suppressed immune systems. This means that the body's immune system that fights off disease-carrying germs and bacteria cannot work properly. If you do not consume and absorb adequate vital nutrients, your immunity cannot be strong. When your immune system is weak, infections take over, and you are more prone to catching colds, flus and viruses. Children who continually suffer colds eventually grow up into adults with potentially compromised immune systems.

My clients who suffered from low immune response and then embarked on a program of algae report fewer colds, quicker recovery periods, and a stronger resistance to catching viruses and flus. This may be due to the algae's rich nutritional profile of minerals, vitamins, enzymes and proteins that are needed for a healthy functioning immune system. Wild blue-green algae also exhibits antimicrobial, antiviral and antibacterial activity. The algae contains high levels of vitamin C and the other antioxidants, vitamin E, selenium, zinc, beta-carotene and nucleic acids. It is speculated that the sulfolipids, vitamin B12 and nucleotides may be the compounds responsible for this activity.

However, it is the high concentration of beta-carotene which activates the thymus gland; the thymus gland can then control the immune system effectively. Beta-carotene greatly enhances the immune system and may inhibit the development of cancer cells.[32] The beta-carotene content within wild blue-green algae is extraordinarily high. Hans Nieper, M.D., the renowned cancer specialist in Germany, recommends beta-carotene to his patients. Charles Simone, M.D., author of *Cancer and Nutrition*, recommends a diet high in beta-carotene, because of the link with inhibiting cancer. Simone states, "Studies done by the US Department of Agriculture Food Intake Survey show that the average American diet provides beta-carotene in amounts that are much less than that recommended to prevent cancer." Dr. Simone claims that beta-carotene blocks the process by which a cell can turn malignant. It should be noted that beta-carotene is extremely safe and non-toxic.[33] Studies on animals, published in the *Journal of the National Cancer Institute*, indicate that beta-carotene increases immune system action against certain forms of cancer cells.[34]

Finally, research findings published in *The Journal of the National Cancer Institute* in 1989 indicated that chemicals derived from blue-green algae inhibited the growth of the AIDS virus.[35]

ACIDIC BODIES

I see many people at my clinic who are suffering from acidosis, a condition in which the body is simply too acidic. If you don't eat enough alkaline-forming foods like fresh fruit, vegetables and salads, you can create an acid stomach. When the body is too acid, it provides a fertile ground for acute and chronic disease. Kidney, liver and adrenal disorders, poor diet, obesity, stress and toxemia can create acidosis. Stress, sugar, animal products, dairy, eggs and even grains might have an acidifying effect on the body. Symptoms of acidosis can include stomach ulcers, insomnia, headaches, gas, bloating, foul-smelling stools, water retention, arthritis and other more serious health problems.

An acid body means that there is an excess of hydrogen ions which combine with oxygen to form water. This excess hydrogen depletes the body's oxygen. Simply stated, a shortage of oxygen causes cells to break down and die, creating acidosis. The more acidic the system, the less the biochemical buffers are able to maintain the blood's healthy acid-alkaline balance. A more serious consequence of acidity is that it causes calcium to be mobilized out of your bones through urine; such conditions create fertile ground for conditions like osteoporosis. Excess acid may also get deposited in cell tissues, eventually causing arthritis. Wild blue-green algae, with its perfect balance of sodium, potassium, calcium and magnesium, can actually reverse an over-acid system.

Acidosis Self-Evaluation

Watch your own acid/alkaline progress as you embark on a blue-green algae program. Buy Nitrazine paper at a drugstore. Apply your urine to the paper either *before* eating or one hour after. The paper will change color to indicate if your system is overly acidic. Once you are regularly taking algae, you could perform this acidosis self-evaluation each week, and hopefully, witness your biochemistry improve.

ANEMIA

Anemia is basically too little blood in the system. This means that there is a reduction in the oxygen-carrying protein of the red blood cells, limiting the amount of oxygen the blood can carry; reduction in the number of red blood cells occurs. Symptoms may include fatigue, dizziness, drowsiness, pale appearance, mouth soreness, constipation, headaches, loss of appetite, irritability, loss of menstrual periods in women. This type of blood deficiency can be caused by a lack of nutrients, poor diet, inability to absorb nutrients, or weak digestion. In order to build blood and prevent anemia, you need enough iron, folic acid, B12, protein, vitamin E, nutrients in abundance in the AFA wild blue-green algae. Iron is an important factor in anemia because iron makes hemoglobin, the protein that carries oxygen to the cells. Wild blue-green algae is the richest known source of assimilable iron and bioavailable minerals needed to ultimately prevent or reverse anemia. In order to absorb iron, you need adequate copper, B vitamins and vitamin C, again all nutrients contained within wild blue-green algae.

On another level, according to Dr. Jonathan Wright, the single most common reason for anemia is a lack of (or low) stomach acid which is needed to absorb iron and B12. Gastric acid secretion is critical to iron absorption and the assimilation of other nutrients. Those who suffer from inferior stomach acid production are often low in zinc and niacin as well. In my own practice, I have found that zinc and niacin absorption is superior when ingesting wild blue-algae, thus positively affecting stomach acid secretions. A lack of vitamin B12, which can also cause a type of anemia, is often due to a defect in absorption, and wild blue-green algae has the richest known source of vitamin B12 in a form that the body can easily use. Folic acid deficiency can also lead to a type of anemia, and the algae is high in assimilable levels of folic acid.

Finally, wild blue-green algae is the richest known source of chlorophyll. Chlorophyll has been used for years to eradicate anemia and enhance blood supply. The chlorophyll molecule in wild blue-green algae is almost identical to the pigment in our human red blood cells. The difference is that chlorophyll contains magnesium at the center, whereas blood contains iron. In laboratory experiments with anemic animals, red blood cell counts have returned to normal within four or five days when chlorophyll was given.[36]

SWEET CRAVINGS—HYPOGLYCEMIA

Wild blue-green algae is ideal for taming that sweet tooth and keeping hypoglycemia under control. (Hypoglycemia is an abnormal low blood sugar concentration, sometimes precipitated by an inadequate diet.) Hypoglycemia may cause the following symptoms: dizziness, headaches, sweet cravings, substance abuse or addictions, irritability, weakness, chest tightness, confusion, anxiety, constant hunger. Hypoglycemia will adversely affect mental processes, since the brain needs adequate blood sugar supply. Proper diet is the key to maintaining balanced sugar levels. Bernard Jensen in his book, *Nature Has a Remedy*, states that hypoglycemic symptoms occur in over half of the American population.

Wild blue-green algae contains a sufficient quantity of predigested carbohydrates to supply energy. The predigested proteins in the algae calm blood sugar fluctuations in both hypoglycemia and hyperglycemia (diabetes). The algae's carbohydrates and proteins are in forms that are easy for the body to assimilate and metabolize. To control a sugar craving, take half a teaspoon of wild blue-green algae powder mixed in water at the time of the craving. This dosage may need to be increased depending on the severity of the symptoms. Wild blue-green algae can help to rebuild the sugar-regulating function of the adrenals, liver and pancreas due to its optimum levels of usable protein. The algae provides its protein in the most usable form, glycoprotein; the body does not need to waste time nor metabolic energy in converting lipoproteins to glycoproteins when algae is ingested. Yet this tiresome conversion may be all too frequent when eating animal or other foods. High-protein diets are often suggested for hypoglycemic individuals. However, protein from meat is not the best source, since too much meat can create an excess of urea or uric acid; a saturation of uric acid weakens the kidneys as it also leaches calcium from the body. Wild blue-green algae is the richest whole food of assimilable protein.

BLEEDING GUMS

I see many people who complain of bleeding gums, either when they floss or simply when they brush their teeth. Bleeding gums or inflamed gums, commonly known as gingivitis, is a sign of an unhealthy mouth and body. *Common causes:* Bacteria, mucus, congestion, accumulation of food particles. Gingivitis, if untreated, can lead to periodontital disease whereby gums swell, seep pus and recede; ultimately, teeth may shift, causing the jawbone to become smaller, and allowing bacterial invasion.

Oral hygiene is important in preventing these mouth problems. However, in every case of gingivitis that I have seen, nutritional deficiencies play a significant role in prevention. Wild blue-green algae has corrected the problem within four to eight weeks depending on severity of symptoms. A lack of vitamin C and E can cause gums to be soft. Deficiencies of calcium, phosphorus, folic acid and niacin can also contribute to gum inflammation and poor bone health. Wild blue-green algae plays a preventative role in the formation of bacteria due to its high chlorophyll content. Because chlorophyll breaks down carbon dioxide and releases free oxygen, it inhibits the action of harmful bacteria; these bacteria cannot flourish in an oxygenated environment. Finally, the high content of beta-carotene, with its anti-infection qualities, contributes to the health of the gums.

SKIN CONDITIONS

I have successfully used wild blue-green algae for patients combating eczema, dermatitis, acne, warts and cold sores. Six months ago, a 17-year-old boy came into my clinic desperate for help. He told me, "None of the girls will go out with me because of my terrible acne." The acne was quite prominent on his face and neck. He had visited several physicians over the past two years who prescribed mostly antibiotics. Nothing happened, except that the teenager did not feel well from the medications. His mother was concerned about the long-term use of these drugs, particularly the antibiotics, both oral and cream, including cortisone. In fact, while on cortisone, the skin condition worsened. Symptoms of flatulence, bloating and constipation appeared.

My program: Gradual build-up to 3 heaping teaspoons of wild blue-green algae powder every day (approximately 6 grams). Wild blue-green algae is rich in GLA essential fatty acids, which can often help to rectify a faulty fat metabolism (the root cause of many skin problems). The high chlorophyll content of the algae helped to purify the blood of the toxins that cause skin eruptions. The vitality of one's skin is often related to the condition of the lungs, kidneys or liver. For example, if your kidneys are congested, it is likely that your skin will appear lifeless, or worse. As a health practitioner, poor skin is a "red flag" for me to check the status of kidneys, lungs or liver. When these organs are overburdened, toxins may secrete through the skin. Molecular properties of wild blue-green algae can protect and restore the liver and kidneys by clearing out the toxins.

The high beta-carotene/provitamin A content of wild blue-green algae is beneficial for skin eruptions, healing damaged tissue and construction of new skin. Vitamin A is critical to the proper development and maintenance of cell tissues; when vitamin A is deficient, skin problems will undoubtedly occur.[37] Other key nutrients critical for the maintenance of healthy skin: zinc, chromium, selenium, vitamin E, pantothenic acid, B vitamins, nucleic acids, vitamin C and niacin; they fight infection, fend off bacteria, flush out toxins and feed skin tissue. All these nutrients are contained in the AFA algae. I also recommend spirulina, propolis, lecithin, hydrochloric acid, specific enzyme preparations and my own edible algae face mask. (See my Face Mask Recipe on page 46.) It is important to eliminate dairy products, chocolate, wheat, sugar, caffeine and alcohol from the diet. The 17-year-old patient followed this treatment exactly, never missing the recommended course of algae. He had also suffered varying allergic reactions to certain foods. He reported to me recently that the food allergies have diminished and his bowels are moving regularly. He now eats lots of raw vegetables, and maintains a dosage of 2 level teaspoons of wild blue-green algae every day (2 grams)) Today, the teenager is acne-free and I am pleased to announce that he got the girl!

ANTI-AGING

Free-radical damage causes premature aging. The antioxidant component of AFA wild blue-green algae can offer some protection. The great quantity of pre-digested digestive enzymes help to improve digestive absorption so that the body cna take up more immune building anti-aging nutrients. The AFA algae's large store of nucleic acids (RNA and DNA) benefit cellular renewal and potentially reverse, or at least slow, the aging process.

WEIGHT LOSS

Wild blue-green algae is the best green superfood to use in cases of obesity or excess weight. I use it in my patients' weight-loss programs. For those with a diet history of meat, dairy, eggs and processed foods, wild blue-green algae can work very well. The fatty acid content and specific amino acids are highly effective for weight reduction. The AFA algae's amino acid protein is easily absorbed by the body; this, along with other compounds, keeps blood glucose levels stable. Since hunger is registered in the brain whenever blood glucose or amino levels are low, keeping these nutrients high can fool the body into thinking it's not hungry. Stabilizing blood sugar levels will keep appetites under control. In addition, the high amino acid content can influence neurotransmitters in the brain, especially those controlling appetite. If you are low in even one amino acid, brain chemistry fluctuations and imbalances will occur. In other words, when using AFA algae as part of a weight-loss program in high enough dosages, you may not feel as hungry, due to very positive biochemical changes. The fatty acid content, broad mineral range and iodine content also help to regulate weight levels. AFA algae can also reduce toxic load and excess fluids in the body, normally associated with overweight problems.

HEAVY METAL POISONING

I frequently encounter clients with high levels of toxic metals in the brain or bloodstream. Excess levels of toxic metals can be absorbed into your system through food, air, water and even teeth fillings. Many weakened conditions can be linked to an overload of toxic metals in the body including Alzheimer's disease, hypertension, kidney, liver and heart problems, as well as central nervous system disorders.

AFA algae stimulates the chelating or discharge of toxic residues, builds up the blood and renews cellular tissue. I have found the most dramatic results using blue-green algae to remove the following:

CADMIUM (can damage the immune system).

LEAD (causes a host of problems from yeast overgrowth, infertility and inability to absorb iron leading to anemia to protein deficiencies and hyperactivity).[38]

MERCURY (accumulates in the brain and central nervous system causing depression, fatigue, dizziness and insomnia).

These toxic metals leach vital minerals from the body. AFA algae also contains certain amino acids which tie up metals like mercury and cadmium, rendering these metals less harmful. Some algae amino acid components counteract toxic molecules to form non-toxic substances which are rapidly excreted in the urine. I recommend approximately 6–10 grams daily for severe cases of metal toxicity. Toxic metal reduction should be carried out under the supervision of a nutritionist or qualified health practitioner.

LIVER FATIGUE

Studies now show that poor diet, stressful lifestyle, medications, alcohol and environmental pollutants cause untold damage to our livers.[39] Energy is diverted from the digestive system, reducing the body's supply of digestive enzymes and decreasing nutrient absorption. End result: digestive disturbances, improper levels of fat, protein and blood sugar, disturbance in neurotransmitters and brain waves, mineral imbalances and liver fatigue. Everyone is at risk of liver fatigue, the swelling or sluggishness of this important organ. Some symptoms of liver fatigue: tumors, growths, tiredness, stress, bloated stomach, menstrual problems, indigestion, skin disorders, swollen glands, a feeling of a lump in your throat, bodily pains and depression. Your liver, the largest organ in your body, needs to be able to process and destroy harmful substances such as drugs, poisons, chemicals, viruses and bacterial infections. The liver stores important nutrients, produces others, and most important, secretes a fluid called bile which is critical for digestion.

AFA algae may be the best natural remedy for combating liver degradation or imbalances. It boasts the highest levels of B12, which protects the liver from injurious toxins. The liver itself is the main storage site for B12; if there is a deficiency, the liver is vulnerable to weakness. AFA algae is also one of the few blue-green algaes which contain choline; a deficiency of choline can cause fatty degeneration of the liver, venous congestion and constipation. AFA contains methionine, an amino acid capable of detoxifying harmful compounds in the liver. The liver also needs high-quality assimilable protein to help fight infection and bacteria. AFA algae contains all eight essential and semiessential amino acids. The amino acid profile is similar to that of the human body, with protein units that are small enough to be directly absorbed into the bloodstream. Arthritis, allergies, anemia, diabetes, hypertension, obesity, alcoholism, infertility, digestive disorders, constipation, toxic metal overload and low energy all should respond favorably to liver cleaning, aided by AFA algae.

The high level of beta-carotene within AFA algae can play a major role in the various processes of the liver. If you consume a diet rich in greasy, preservative-laden, highly processed foods, you will undoubtedly overwork your liver and cause a beta-carotene deficiency. However, by consuming AFA algae, a beta-carotene deficiency is almost impossible. You may find that by using this algae for liver protection, you will improve your eyes as well. The high levels of AFA-source beta-carotene can benefit the eyes, simultaneously helping the liver. Red eyes, inflamed eyes, glaucoma, cataracts and visual abnormalities basically mirror the condition of the liver, and can all be improved with a program of this algae. Biotin, inositol, vitamin C and other concentrated liver-supporting nutrients are all contained in wild blue-green algae. Finally, AFA algae contains the blue pigment phycocyanin, a compound similar to the human pigment bilirubin found in the liver; this substance is essential for proper liver function and the digestion of amino acids. If you suffer from liver fatigue, you should benefit from the standard dosages of AFA algae (2 grams daily).

DEPRESSION

Mental depression is often caused by a stagnant liver accompanied by a host of nutritional deficiencies; virtually *any* nutrient deficiency can result in depression. Wild blue-green algae has an antidepressant action. The reason that AFA works so well to lift mood is that it is high in the nutrients that seem to be the most common deficiencies in depressed people. For example, folic acid (folate) deficiency is the most common nutrient deficiency. Many studies have shown severely depressed individuals to be folate deficient. Low levels of B1 (thiamine) are also common, resulting in body acidosis and altered brain chemistry. AFA is high in B1 and folate. B6 levels and niacin are also typically low in depressed individuals, especially those on oral contraceptive pills.[40] AFA contains adequate levels of these key nutrients. Finally, specific amino acids, which can alter brain chemistry, are present in the proper balance in AFA algae. This helps to prevent brain chemistry fluctuations which could cause emotional or psychological imbalances. I have found AFA to be a true brain "elixir" and mood elevator. Two grams of wild blue-green algae 2–3 times daily might do the trick when feeling tired, depressed or blue.

ANTIBIOTICS

Long-term use of antibiotics has a detrimental effect on the human body. According to Dr. Remy Chauvin of the Sorbonne, Paris, "The overuse of antibiotics is causing unhealthy bacteria to develop marked resistance." Many viral bacteria are on a dramatic increase because they are becoming immune to the drugs. To complicate this process, the drugs destroy the good, healthy "friendly bacteria" in the gut. This means that your body can no longer effectively produce certain vitamins and digestive enzymes, since healthy intestinal flora are destroyed. A compromised intestinal tract will not maintain a high concentration of vitamins or healthy bacteria. Wild blue-green algae can help to restore the delicate balance of healthy intestinal flora, and replenish nutrients lost from an antibiotic onslaught.

Case Study synopsis: Young girl, 10
Symptoms: 10 months of pussing spots all over trunk of body, neck and arm. She had been on several courses of antibiotic drugs to no avail. The doctors could not find anything wrong. Blood tests at my clinic revealed mineral deficiencies across the board, including zinc, calcium and magnesium. Her body pH was acidic. Feeling tired and lethargic. After 4 weeks of algae, pussing spots had started to disappear; after 8 weeks, pussing spots mostly disappeared; after 10 weeks, completely cleared up. Child more energized, happy.

MUCUS CONGESTION

An excess of pollutants, pollens, dirt, dust, debris, germs, bacteria, cigarette smoke, and other unwanted substances can cause the overproduction of heavy, unhealthy (and usually unpleasant) mucus. This heavy mucus production or catarrh often leads to (or may be the result of) allergies or sensitivities, asthma, inflammation, bronchitis, sinusitis, emphysema and immune system dysfunction. The wild blue-green AFA algae helps to dry excess mucus, neutralize allergic responses, and act as an anti-inflammatory agent for inflamed passageways. My clients, who originally came to me with mucus congestion, tell me that they can breathe better since being on the algae program; they seem to have fewer allergies. The AFA wild blue-green algae has a powerful effect on the immune system, boosting nutrient load, freeing the liver of toxins, and reducing allergic responses.

Clinical Case Study: Beverley, Patient, 42

Recently, a 42-year-old opera singer came to my clinic. She told me that I was her last resort, and that her career as an international opera star "will not survive" unless she gets help. Two years ago, she suffered a nasty bout of flu and laryngitis. She was prescribed a long course of antibiotics and cortisone injections for her inflamed tonsils. Since that time, she has suffered with perpetual lingering sore throats. The throat problems inhibited her ability to sing well. She also complained that her nasal passages felt blocked. She had an opera performance coming up in six weeks and was already in rehearsals. As time was of the essence, I took the most aggressive approach possible. Over a four-week period, we built up to two heaping teaspoons of wild blue-green algae powder twice daily. For the first week of the algae introduction, my opera diva lived on a mucus-free diet: only ingesting blended fruits, vegetable juices and broths.

Patient noticed a marked difference after only one week, but was afraid to get too excited for fear that her sore throat would return. My aggressive treatment was continued throughout her rehearsal period plus the month of opera concerts. The blue-green algae opened up her clogged nasal passages, and acted as a natural antiviral agent, fighting microbes and viruses in her body. The bioflavonoid enzymes and PABA in the algae helped to block the building of prostaglandins, the fat compounds that cause symptoms of pain and inflammation of mucous membranes. My opera singer patient now reports no throat soreness, and was just offered a starring role in yet another major opera production.

Comment: The only concern about such an aggressive approach with the algae is that there is the potential for a "cleaning-out response"—a high dosage may cause excessive release of bowel movements, or in some cases, diarrhea.

BOWEL MOVER AND MILD DIURETIC

Miss T., a well-known television actress, was totally blocked when she first came to see me. She had never moved her bowels regularly, suffering from constipation since childhood. She sometimes did not move her bowels for up to six days! She suffered from fluid retention in her ankles. Stool tests revealed a major imbalance of gut flora, and some pathogenic bacteria. Blood results revealed low magnesium, folic acid and iron, which also can contribute to poor elimination and constipation. Her tongue often appeared sore, with a dark red coloring and thick coating. This suggested to me that her liver was stagnant with reduced energy flow through the gastrointestinal areas. Her bowel movements were usually dry and hard, indicating a "hot" or inflamed liver; liver inflammation is frequently the result of poor diet exacerbated by poor elimination. This type of liver stagnancy reduces peristalsis, the wavelike muscular contraction of the intestines. Result: delayed bowel movements.

I started Miss T. on a gentle program of blue-green algae.

Week 1:	¼ teaspoon
Week 2:	½ teaspoon mixed with aloe vera juice
Week 3:	¾ teaspoon
Week 4:	1 teaspoon

First, wild blue-green algae has a very mild diuretic action, thus reducing the fluid retention in Miss T. Second, the algae has a cooling effect on the body. It won't make you cold, but it encourages the body to contract, pushing the energy lower down. The algae will consequently cool the heat in the liver. Third, its bitter action affects the intestines and increases muscle contractions and peristalsis, resulting in more efficient bowel movements. Miss T. now moves her bowels every day, usually twice daily. (It is best to move your bowels at least two or three times every day.) Miss T's mineral levels and gut flora have normalized. She reports an abundant increase of mental energy. Wild blue-green algae will be useful for inflammations, infections, constipation, fluid retention, swellings, sores, rashes and eruptions. The body's life energy and fluids are directed inward and downward by ingesting the algae. I would go so far as to postulate that even anger and aggression may be reduced since these emotions are also linked to blockages in the human system.

Comment: Proper bowel elimination rids the body of toxins and bacteria, ultimately helping you to feel well. The average healthy person ought to move the bowels 2 to 3 times each day. In fact, new research suggests that infrequent or incomplete bowel elimination may result in an array of ailments including diabetes mellitus, meningitis, myasthenia gravis, thyroid disease, ulcerative colitis, just to name a few.[41]

CANDIDIASIS

When I was younger, I suffered for many years from a variety of symptoms, including chronic exhaustion, migraine headaches, menstrual pains, memory loss, sinus congestion, digestive problems, flu-like symptoms and extreme chemical sensitivity. My ill health began in my teens with a bout of glandular fever, treated by a course of antibiotics. It worsened over the years and eventually a brain tumor was suspected, and an appointment made for a brain scan.

Three days before the scheduled scan, a remarkable "spiritual healer," Marian Moore of Philadelphia, "read" me and diagnosed a severe allergy to yeast and molds—which tests confirmed conclusively, showing a severe overgrowth of the yeast *Candida albicans*.

Candida albicans is a yeast-like fungus that breeds in the intestinal tract, throat, mouth or genitalia. This fungus is supposed to live in a healthy balance within our bodies, but certain internal or external conditions may cause it to multiply out of control, (a condition known as candidiasis): for example, antibiotics, prescription medications, surgery, stress and poor diet. Yeast overgrowth weakens the immune system, as it causes a multitude of possible symptoms including gastrointestinal upset, bloating, itching rectum, gas, constipation, stomach cramps, sore throat, allergies, nasal and sinus congestion, facial pain, vaginal infections, nausea, depression, weight problems, hives, earaches and of course, migraine headaches. In my own case, Candida and a host of adverse bacteria were growing out of control in my digestive tract, bloodstream, intestinal lining and other tissues. My body was, in essence, poisoning itself. As a result, I was unable to absorb vitamins, minerals or amino acids.

Ailments such as candidiasis, viral infections, parasites, pathogens, sinusitis, edema, tumors, arthritis, multiple sclerosis and even cancer are all associated with what I call "damp conditions." Dampness, often in the initial form of mucus congestion, ultimately affects the heart, lungs, liver, kidneys, digestion and other bodily functions and organs. The solution to these damp conditions is to dry the excess fluids and drain the dampness. Changing the diet and food intake is certainly helpful, but it alone will *not* arrest the damp condition and associated symptoms or ailments. Instead, I have developed a program rotation of powerful herbal fungicides accompanied by 10 grams a day of the AFA wild blue-green algae. This has proven to be a most powerful remedy, especially in light of the fact that yeasts and other bacterias are now often immune to antibiotics. The AFA algae essentially dries the excess fluids and helps to drain the dampness.[42] This is the first critical step to ultimate wellness.

DOSAGES

Your introduction to wild blue-green algae should begin slowly. This potent food is new to your body; your system may need time to adjust to its effects. It is best to start with the minimum dosage and increase it according to your needs. You may need to do some experimenting, or better yet, consult a qualified nutritionist or informed health practitioner. Various factors will influence dosage requirements: level of activity, degree of imbalances and deficiencies, weight and general health. The correct dosage level should result in more energy and fewer cravings. Some may notice an increase in physical and mental energy quite early in the program. Correct dosages can span a wide range. I have patients on dosages ranging from 2–10 grams daily, depending upon personal symptoms and specific biochemical needs.

In very general terms, I recommend gradually working up to approximately two teaspoons every day for the best, long-term results. But everyone's biochemistry is different. Listen to your body, as some may need higher dosages for best results; some may require lower dosages. Small amounts can still make a big difference in the way you feel.

The more unbalanced or toxic the person is, the less algae should be taken at the beginning. For rejuvenating or detoxifying the liver, or for decreasing other major symptoms, plan on taking algae for at least a year. You may notice an increase in physical and mental energy quite early in an algae ingestion program. If you do not feel any difference in your health, you may be taking too little or you may already be at optimum health. Stress can cause a depletion of important nutrients in the body. During stressful times, you may need more algae (4–10 grams daily). Taking the algae at different times of the day can be a helpful boost. Some people taking the algae for the first time may experience an adverse reaction, for example, a mild frontal headache or possibly diarrhea; it usually indicates a beneficial healing reaction, although in some cases, too much is being taken. The headache or diarrhea may be due to an adjustment of glucose metabolism. Eating complex carbohydrates should relieve the symptom. In either case, take less for a couple of weeks. Gradually increase the dosage again. Although it is preferable to take algae on an empty stomach or before meals, eating algae after meals or at mealtimes can often reduce any unpleasant reactions when introducing this new food into your diet. If you are already pregnant, it is best to wait until after you deliver your baby before you introduce algae to your diet.

However, if you are thinking of trying to conceive, then it is best to begin an algae program *before* getting pregnant (six months to a year prior to conception). In this way, the body has the proper time to adjust to the new algae regime.

With chronic arthritis, take small dosages in the beginning. Increase gradually as microalgae may initially increase pain as toxins are moved out of the system. Similarly, if you suffer chronic intestinal symptoms, you may actually experience additional flatulence at the outset of the program. Microalgae may initially increase fermentation in the gut as it destroys noxious bacteria. This flatulence will subside.[43] (Special note for men only: an algae regimen may enhance sperm count, potency and endurance.)

Algae can often have a strong cleansing and detoxification action when first introduced to your system. Therefore, I recommend a slow build-up, as follows:

Powders:

Week 1:	¼ tsp	daily	1 tsp = approx. 1 gram
Week 2:	½ tsp	daily	
Week 3:	¾ tsp	daily	Mix powders in large
Week 4:	1 tsp	daily	glass of water or juice
Week 5:	1½ tsp	daily	
Week 6:	2 tsp	daily	

Capsules or tablets:

Week 1:	1 daily	4 capsules = approx. 1 gram
Week 2:	2 daily	
Week 3:	3 daily	
Week 4:	5 daily	

Tablets could be chewed for best absorption and results.
Drink 1 large glass of water after taking tablets or capsules.

Liquid:

Week 1:	1 full dropper	Standard dosage = 2–4 full droppers
Week 2:	2 full droppers	
Week 3:	3 full droppers	Mix drops in large glass of water or juice
Week 4:	4 full droppers	

Remember, however, that these are very general recommendations as a basic guideline only; each person's biochemistry, deficiencies, imbalances and lifestyle is so different and may require completely different dosages.

CONCLUSION

Wild blue-green AFA algae is a superb natural source of nutrients for the body. It boasts outstanding levels of chlorophyll, vitamin B12, beta-carotene, iron, protein and many more complementary nutrients in a completely assimilable form. As a result, it can help to increase energy, correct imbalances, oxygenate cells and realize high levels of physical and mental health.

Wild blue-green algae has properties which can aid in alleviating various symptoms and illnesses. As a bitter substance, it influences the heart and mind, helping to clean out mucus accumulations from the arteries, thus stabilizing blood pressure. The bitterness can also help to focus the mind and improve concentration. As a drying substance, AFA algae can remove excessive mucosal moisture from tissues, rendering these cells a less favorable environment for viruses, bacterias, parasites and fungi. Yeasts, tumor or cyst growths, excess phlegm, abscesses, swellings, edema and skin eruptions, all might respond well to programs of AFA algae. It has also been used for patients suffering from cancer, AIDS, Epstein-Barr virus, MS and rheumatoid arthritis where internal "wet conditions" exist. The algae also acts as a coolant, thus relieving constipation, inflammations, infections and fevers. Wild blue-green algae is a neurostimulant, feeding the pathways to the brain. The algae makes amino acids readily available to the brain, thereby stimulating neurotransmitters for improved mental acuity and memory. Excellent results have been observed in preventing the progression of Alzheimer's disease. Wild blue-green is an antidepressant and mood elevator. Mental depression can often be linked to a stagnant liver; AFA can help to overcome liver stagnancy caused by poor diet. This blue-green algae can help to change the body from a state of acidosis to a more alkaline base; in other words, it can purify the blood. A toxic bloodstream can result in acne, boils, eczema, allergies, and ultimately acidosis. When the blood is not healthy, degenerative diseases like cancer and arthritis can gain a grip on your body. The algae also acts as a mild diuretic, reducing water retention, simultaneously removing residues of toxic metals from the body and cleaning lymph fluid. Finally, AFA algae is a relaxant. Its predigested proteins and complex carbohydrates maintain balanced blood sugar levels, supplying energy that lasts.

Aphanizemenon flos-aqua blue-green algae can benefit almost everyone. If you have grown up on meat and potatoes, eggs, dairy products, salty foods, chemically preserved foods, sugary foods, then AFA algae is for you. If you eat on the run, need to lose weight, feel tired, have poor nutritional habits, then this algae is also for you. Even if you think you are the most healthy of specimens, I still recommend the AFA algae. It is a complete source of wholesome nutrients in a world where our foods are so nutrient depleted. It rejuvenates your lungs, purifies the kidneys and feeds the gastrointestinal tract. Wild blue-green algae is a true builder of your body, an amazing cleaner and blood purifier. AFA wild blue-green algae may be more bioavailable than any other natural food source or food supplements. This means that the algae, because of its delicate balance, can assimilate, absorb, digest, metabolize and nutrify in perfect harmony for maximum beneficial results.

DR. MCKEITH'S ALGAE RECIPES

Dr. McKEITH'S ALGAE SALAD DRESSING

4 ounces olive oil, walnut or sesame oil
1 teaspoon sesame seeds
2 teaspoons soy sauce
1 clove finely chopped garlic
1 teaspoon honey
2 teaspoons pure lemon juice or freshly squeezed lemon

2 teaspoons algae powder (or open 2 capsules of algae)
cup of finely chopped raw dill herb (or dill powder)
Sprinkle of salt

Mix in ordinary blender or simply stir with spoon. Enjoy! Blue-green algae powder can also be mixed into guacamole or sprinkled on top of avocado slices as a decorative condiment.

Dr. McKEITH'S ENERGIZER

(You will need a juicer)
4–6 carrots
¼-inch fresh ginger root (approximate size of a thumbnail)

Sprig of parsley
2 capsules blue-green algae powder

Stuff all ingredients through the juicer and enjoy.

Dr. McKEITH'S EDIBLE ALGAE FACE MASK

This is my very own beauty treatment. Made with easily accessible ingredients, this paste is packed with natural nutrients.

2 teaspoons algae powder (or open 2 capsules)
4 tbsp. of virgin olive oil
Half a very soft avocado (crush to a paste)
3 teaspoons pure honey
1 teaspoon pure lemon juice (or freshly squeezed)

1 egg white
4 teaspoons of pure vitamin E oil (or open 4 capsules)
2 teaspoons of pure vitamin A oil (or open 2 capsules)
3 teaspoons aloe vera gel

Thoroughly mash the avocado and vigorously mix in all other ingredients to form a creamy paste. Apply externally to your face and leave for one hour. *Voilà*—your skin might even feel like a baby's bottom! And because the ingredients are so pure and natural, feel free to eat any leftovers. Store in refrigerator if necessary; but use within 24 hours for most advanced nutrification.

My face mask is especially good for sensitive or allergic skins as well. My homemade face mask is an excellent alternative to commercial mass-market brands. Commercial brands often contain perfumes or chemicals which may clog the pores, cause allergic reactions or simply damage skin cell tissue. The bliss of my recipe is that it is cheap and easy to make with easily bought ingredients; and it is good for you too.

ALGAE BATH

Fill bath with water
Add 15 drops of lavender

2 tablespoons algae powder

Enjoy and your pores will soak up the minerals!

HEALTHY HAIR AND SCALP

2 heaping teaspoons of blue-green algae powder
2 tablespoons olive oil

2 tablespoons aloe vera gel
10 drops essential fatty acid liquid

Mix together and massage into scalp.
Apply hot, wet towel.
Leave on for 15 minutes. Shampoo well. This tonic helps to nourish, nutrify and mineralize scalp and hair.

BANISH BLOCKED BOWELS

1. *Upon waking in the morning, mix and drink the following:*
   ¾ cup warm water
   1 level teaspoon blue-green algae
   powder
   ¼ cup of aloe vera juice

   ½ teaspoon spirulina
   4 drops liquid chlorophyll
   (add some pure fruit juice for flavor
   if necessary)

   or:

2. *Mix:*
   1 tablespoon flaxseeds in 2 table-
   spoons warm water

   Allow to stand overnight. It will
   become soft and jello like.

In the morning, add ½ teaspoon of algae powder and 1 tablespoon water. Mix and drink.

ENDNOTES

1. Barry, Dr William, *The Astonishing, Magnificent, Delightful Algae,* Graphic Press: Klamath Falls, Oregon. p.1.
2. Cousins, Gabriel, MD, "Microalgae, First and Finest Superfood," *Body Mind Spirit,* April-May 1995. p.13.
3. Michael, John, "Wild Blue-Green Algae: From Power to Promise," Article, 1995. p.20–24.
4. Fay, Peter, *The Blue-Greens (Cyanophyta-Cyanobacteria).* The Institute of Biology's Studies in Biology, no. 160: Westfield College, University of London, Edward Arnold: London, 1983. pp.1–3.
5. France, Richard, *The Miracle of Super Blue-Green Algae,* Colorado Springs, Colorado, 1994. p.39.
6. Apsley, Dr John W. II, *The Genesis Effect,* Volume I. "Spearheading Regeneration of Wild Blue-Green Algae," Genesis Communications: 1995. p.49.
7. Cousins, Gabriel, *Spiritual Nutrition and the Rainbow Diet,* Cassandra Press: San Rafael, CA, 1986. p.212.
8. Barry, *op.cit.* p.23.
9. Personal communication between author and Dr. Barry.
10. Personal communication between author and Dr. Barry.
11. Whitney & Rolfes, *Understanding Nutrition,* West Publishing Co., Minneapolis/ St. Paul, 1993. pp.406–408.
12. R. Beach "Modern Miracle Men," 74th Congress, 2nd Session US Senate Document No.264, June 1, 1936. US Government Printing Office, Washington DC 1941, p.1. 1936 Government report.
13. Rogers, Sherry, *Tired or Toxic, A Blueprint for Health,* Prestige Publishing: Syracuse, NY, 1990. pp.154–155.

14. Rogers, *op.cit.* p.154.
15. R.J. Cousins and J.M. Hempe, "Zinc," in *Present Knowledge in Nutrition*, 6th Edition, ed. M.L. Brown (Washington D.C: International Life Sciences Institute, Nutrition Foundation, 1990), pp.251–260.
16. C.L. Keen, "Zinc Deficiency and Immune Function," *Annual Review of Nutrition* 10 (1990): 415–431.
17. "Nature's Most Perfect Food," *Creative Living*, August 1990, p.19.
18. Bell, L.S., Fairchild, M.J. *American Dietetic Association*, 1987; 87; 341.
19. Pitchford, Paul, *Healing with Whole-Foods*, North Atlantic Books, Berkeley, CA, 1993. p.191.
20. Howell, Edward, *Enzyme Nutrition*, Avery Publishing Group: Garden City Park, NY, 1985. p.29.
21. Wigmore, Ann, *The Hippocrates Diet and Health Program*, Avery: Wayne, NJ, 1984. p.89.
22. Lee, Lita, *Earthletter*, Vol.1, No.2. Redwood City, CA, June 1991. p.1.
23. Whitaker, Julian, *Health & Healing*, April 1996, Volume 6, No.4. pp.1–2.
24. Troxler, R. and Saffer, B. Harvard School of Dental Medicine, "Algae Derived Phycocanin," Ass. Dental Research General Session 1987 Paper.
25. Pitchford, *op.cit.* p.206.
26. Pitchford, *op.cit.* p.207.
27. France, *op.cit.* p.37.
28. *The Nicaragua Report*, Sevilla, Irma and Aguirre, Nereyda, May 1995. Universidad Centroamericana, Facultad de Ciencias Agropecuarias, Nicaragua: Cell Tech, 1995. p.5.
29. "Green Giants—Ancient Algae and Modern Cereal Grasses," "Spirulina: Heavenly Nutrient," *Delicious:* July/August 1990, p.34–35.
30. March, David, "The Secret Superfood," *Healthy Eating*, 1994. p.43.
31. Studies with author's own patients.
32. Seifter, E. Rettura, G., Seiter, J. et al., "Thymotropic action of Vitamin A," Fed.Proc. 1973, 32, p.947. Simone, *op.cit.* p.75.
33. Bendick, A, "Safety of Beta-Carotene," *Review, Nutr.Cancer* 11:207–214, 1988.
34. Asgiersson, G., Bellanti, J.A. "Exercises, Immunity and Infection," *Sem.Adolescent Med.* 1987, p.31.
35. *Journal of National Cancer Institute*, April 19, 1989, Vol.81, No.8. p.1254–58.
36. *Health Store News*, Rolling Press, Ref. File #010–189–799.
37. Zile, M.H. and Cullum, M.E. "The Function of Vitamin A: Current Concepts," *Proc.Soc. Exp.Biol.Med.*, 1983, 172, pp.139–52.
38. E.R. Monsen, "Iron Nutrition and Absorption: Dietary Factors Which Impact Iron Bioavailability," *Journal of the American Dietetic Association* 88 (1988): 786–790.
39. Viktor Kubinskas, *Survival into the 21st Century*, Woodstock Valley, Connecticut: 21 Century Publications, 1975. pp.24–26.
40. Russ, C., Hendricks, T., Chomley, B., Kalin, N. and Driskell, J., "Vitamin B6 Status of Depressed and Obsessive-Compulsive Patients," *Nutr. Rep. Intl.*, 1983.
41. Murray, Michael & Pizzorno, Joseph, *An Encyclopedia of Natural Medicine*, Prima Publishing: Rocklin, CA, 1991, p.232.
42. Pitchford, *op.cit.* p.59.
43. Holmes, P. *The Energetics of Western Herbs*, p.351.